MY STRENGTH IS YOUR STRENGTH JOURNAL

WINNING AGAINST BREAST CANCER

By Valeda Keys

My Strength is Your Strength

Printed in the United States of America

ISBN: 9781797422268

PREFACE

Use this journal to capture your thoughts, fears, hopes and dreams. May it encourage you to write your journey, whatever it may be. Your story matters. Your thoughts matter. Your desires matter. Your hope matters. Your concerns matter. Your vision matters. And most importantly, YOU matter!

My Strength Is Your Strength.

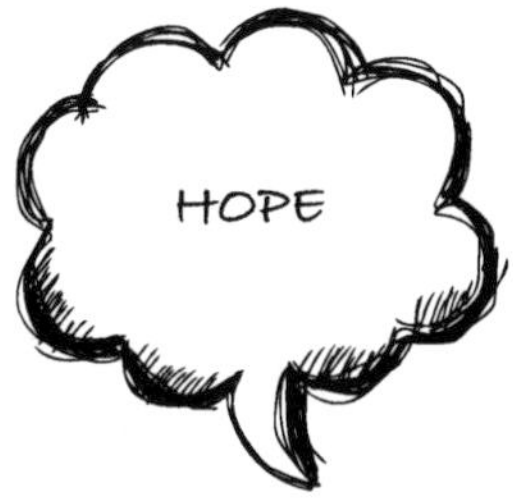
HOPE

MY STRENGTH IS ...

MY **STRENGTH IS ...** ______

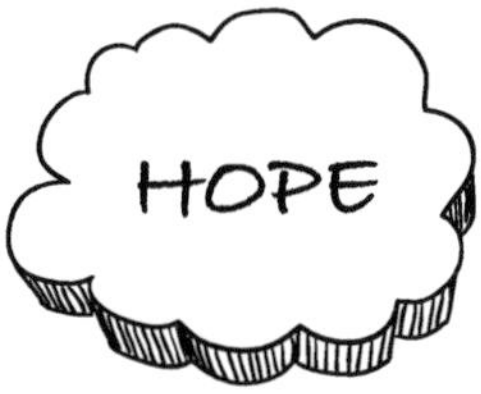
HOPE

MY STRENGTH IS ... ______

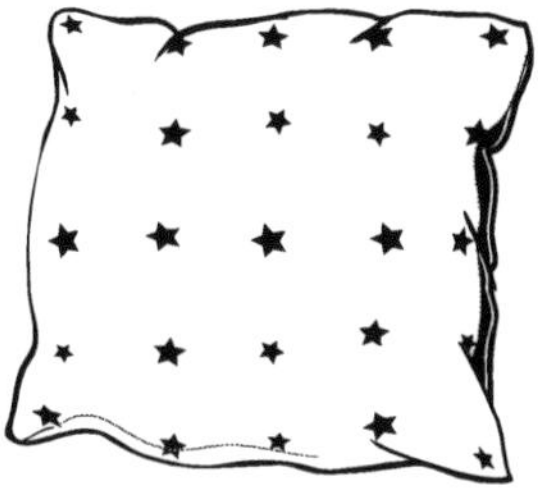

MY STRENGTH IS ...

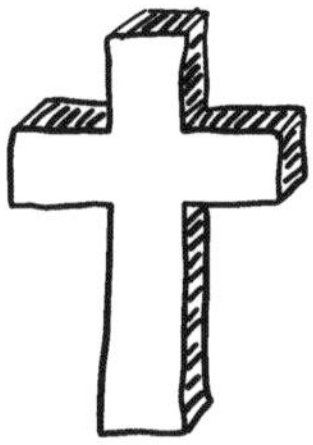

MY STRENGTH IS ...

MY STRENGTH IS ... ______

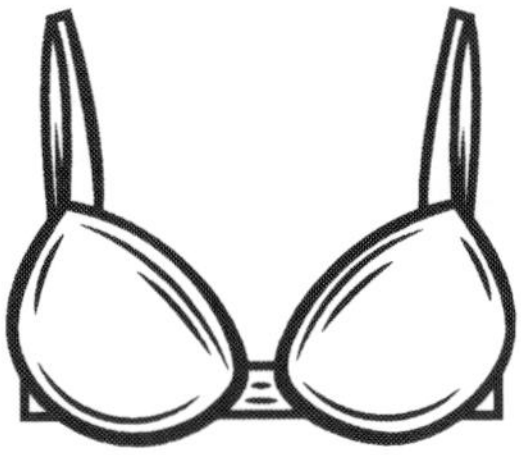

MY STRENGTH IS ...

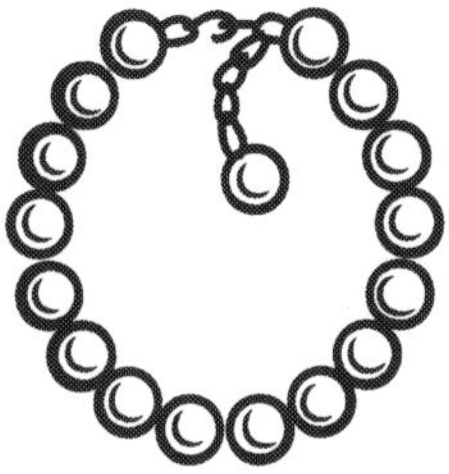

MY STRENGTH IS ... ______________________________

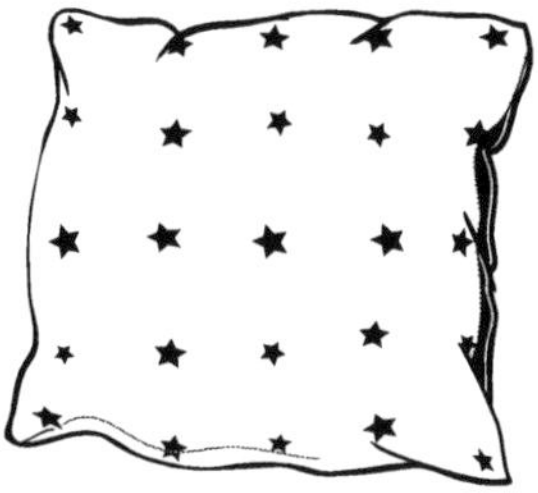

MY STRENGTH IS ... ___

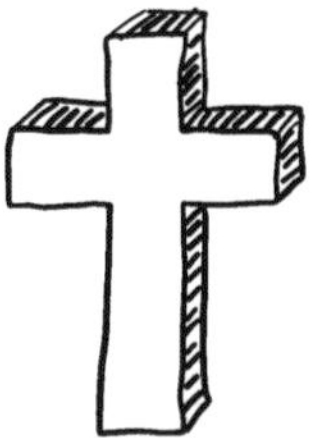

MY STRENGTH IS ... ______

MY STRENGTH IS ...

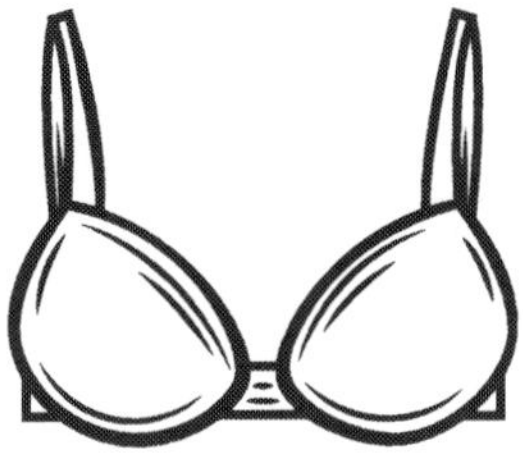

MY STRENGTH IS ... ______

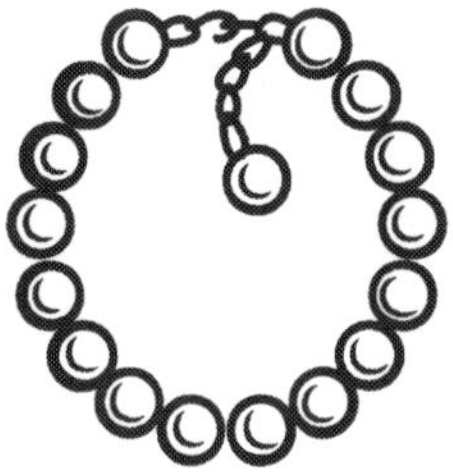

MY STRENGTH IS ... ______

MY STRENGTH IS ... ______________________________

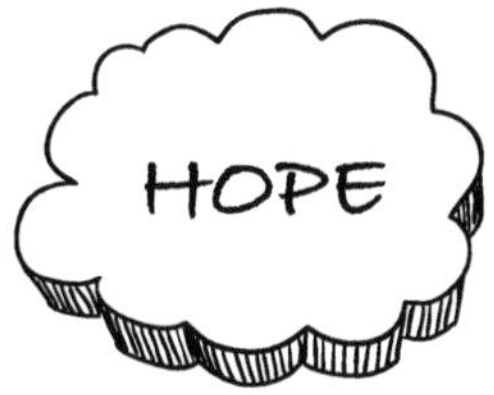
HOPE

MY
STRENGTH IS ... ____

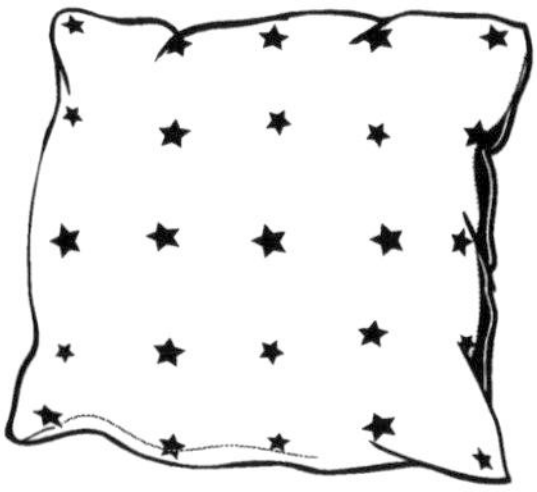

MY STRENGTH IS ...

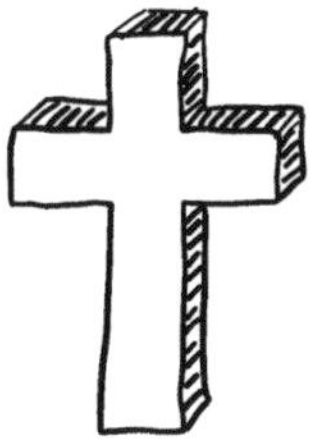

MY STRENGTH IS ...

MY STRENGTH IS ... ____________________

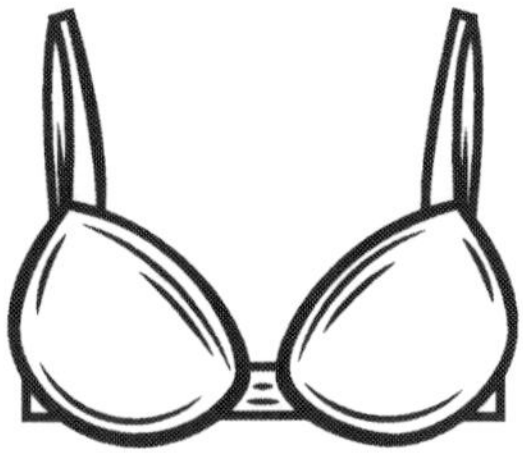

MY STRENGTH IS ...

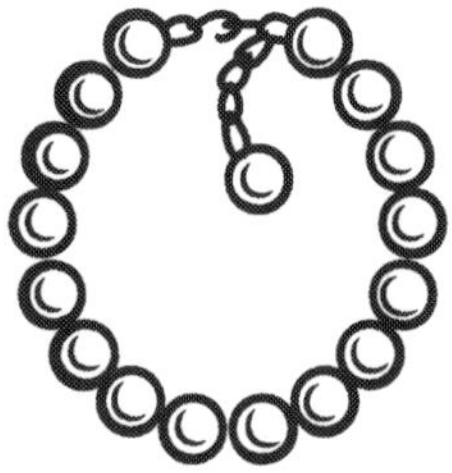

MY STRENGTH IS ...

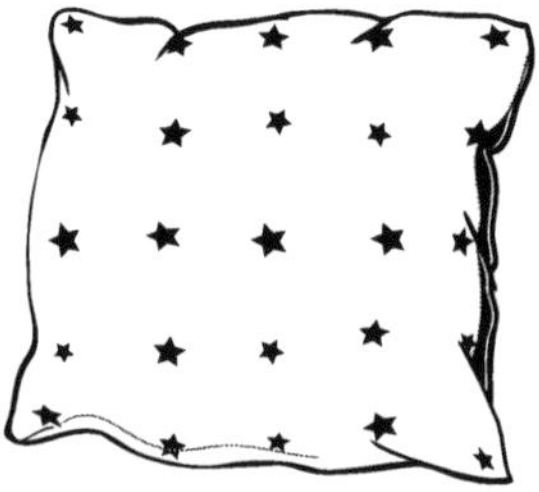

MY STRENGTH IS ... ______

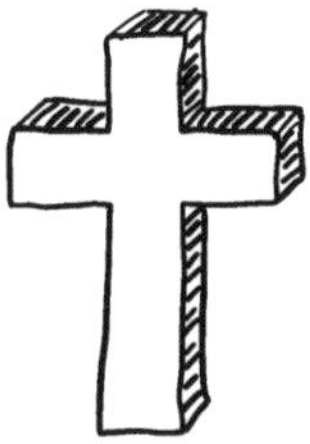

MY STRENGTH IS ... ______________________

MY STRENGTH IS ...

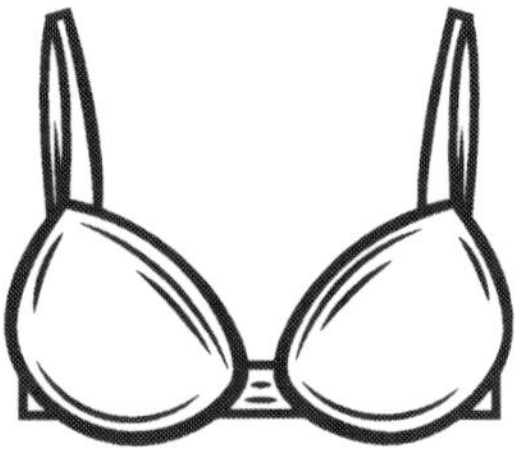

MY STRENGTH IS ... ______________________

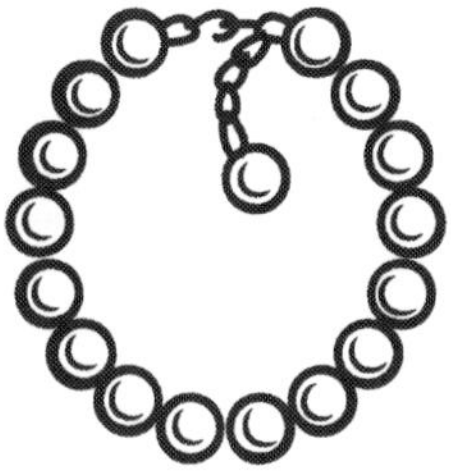

MY STRENGTH IS ...

MY STRENGTH IS ...

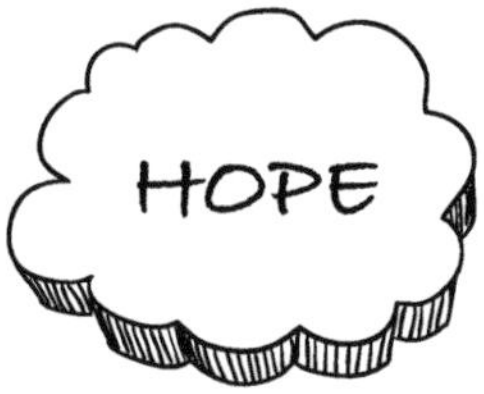
HOPE

MY STRENGTH IS ...

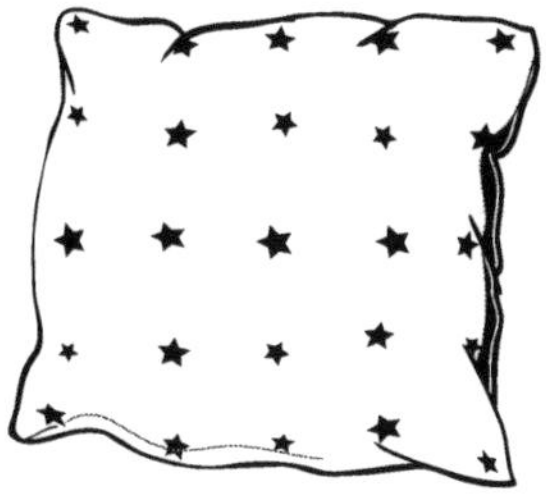

MY STRENGTH IS ...

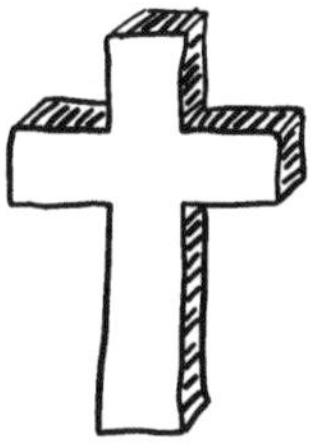

MY STRENGTH IS ...

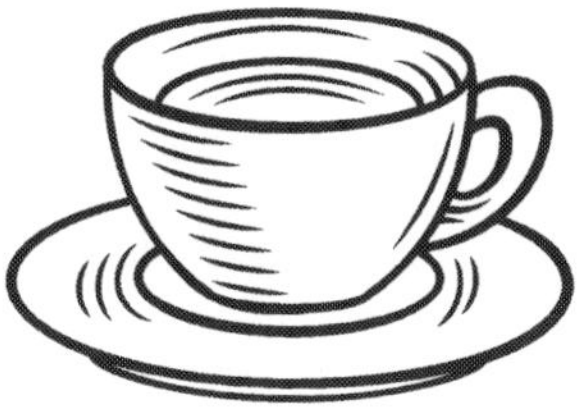

MY STRENGTH IS ...

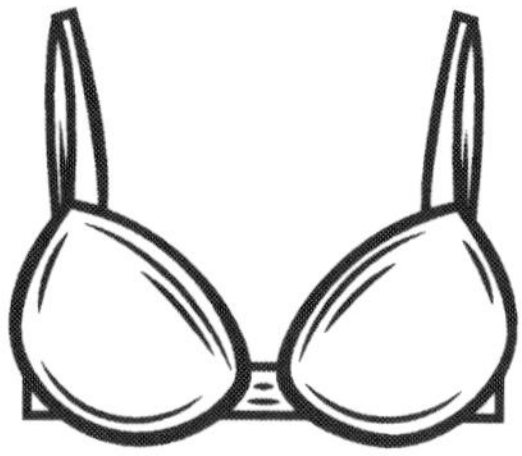

MY STRENGTH IS ...

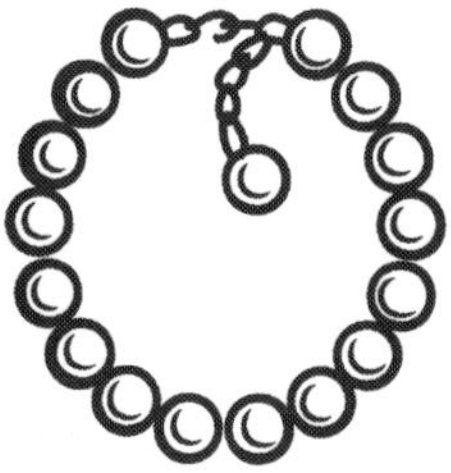

MY STRENGTH IS ...

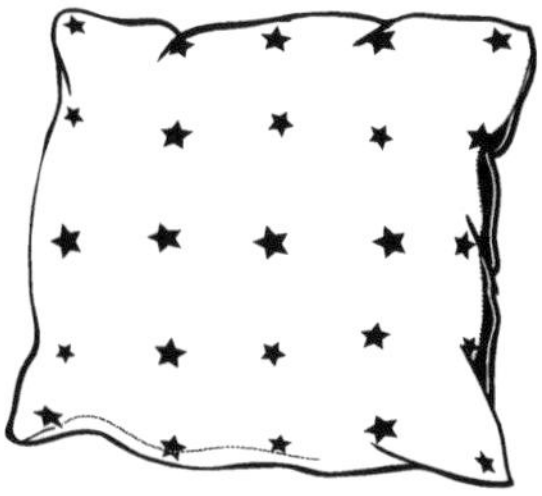

MY STRENGTH IS ... ______

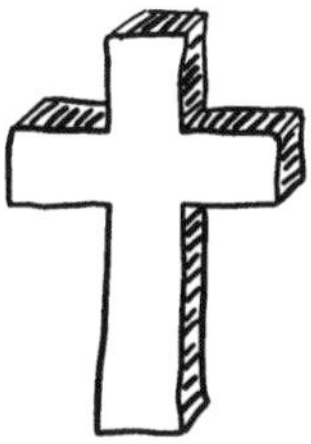

MY STRENGTH IS ...

MY STRENGTH IS ...

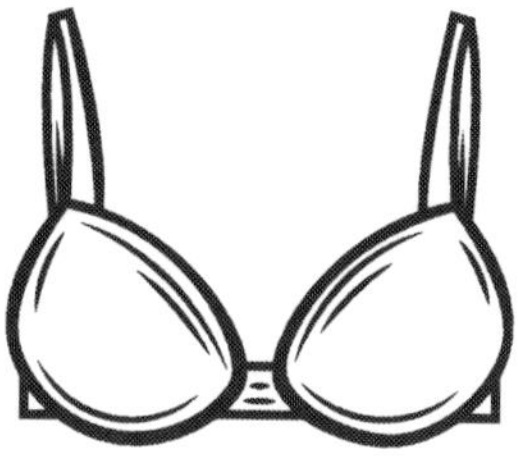

MY STRENGTH IS ...

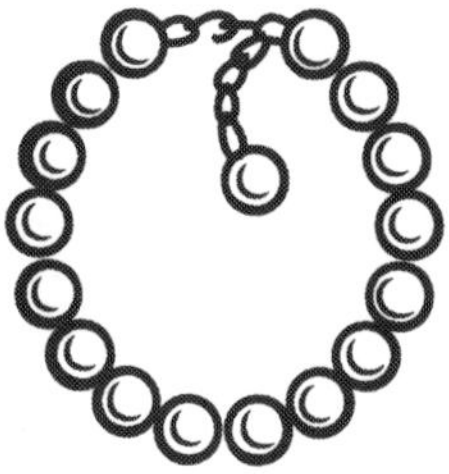

MY STRENGTH IS ...

MY STRENGTH IS ...

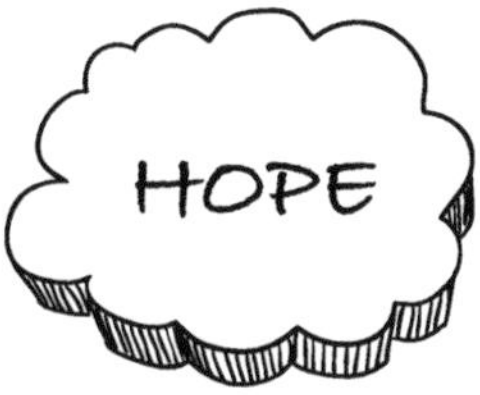
HOPE

MY STRENGTH IS ...

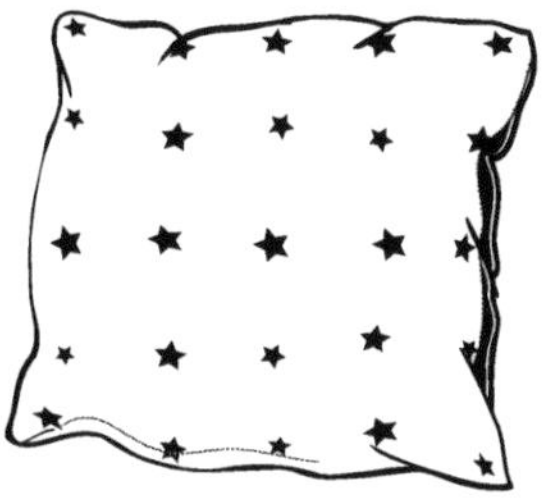

MY STRENGTH IS ...

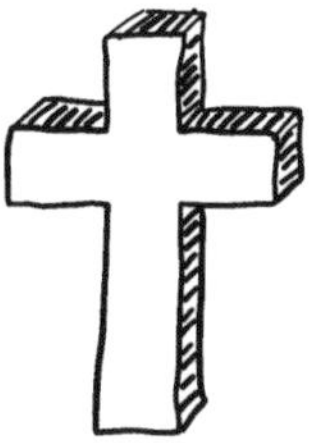

MY STRENGTH IS ...

MY STRENGTH IS ...

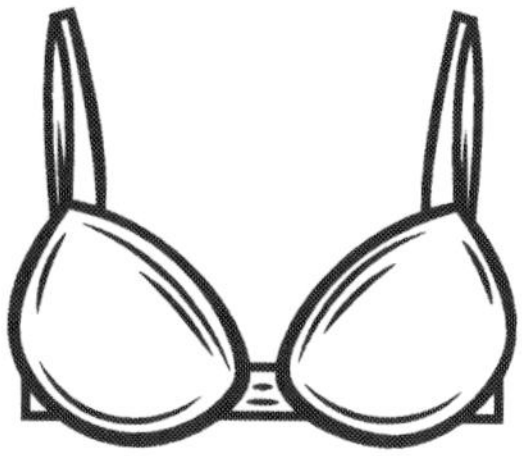

MY STRENGTH IS ...

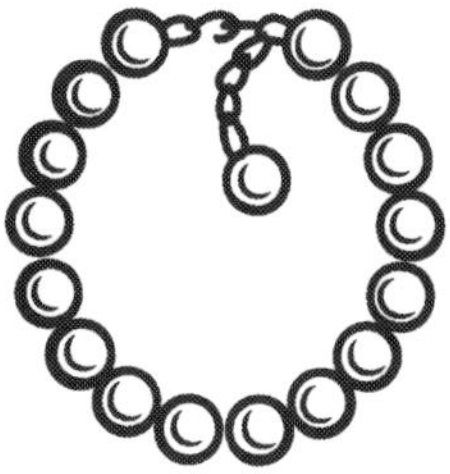

MY
STRENGTH IS ...

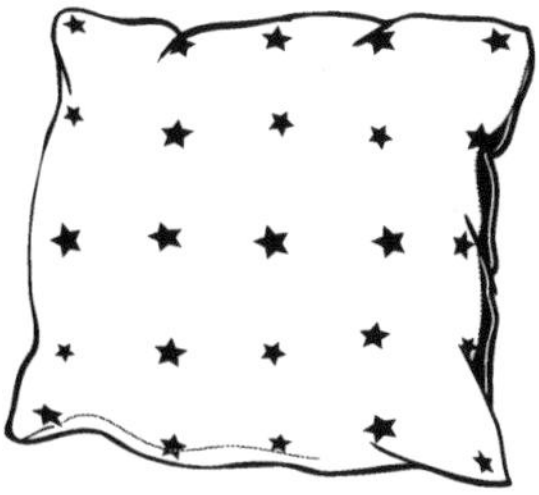

MY STRENGTH IS ...

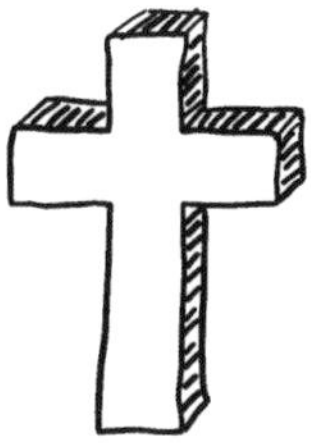

MY STRENGTH IS ...

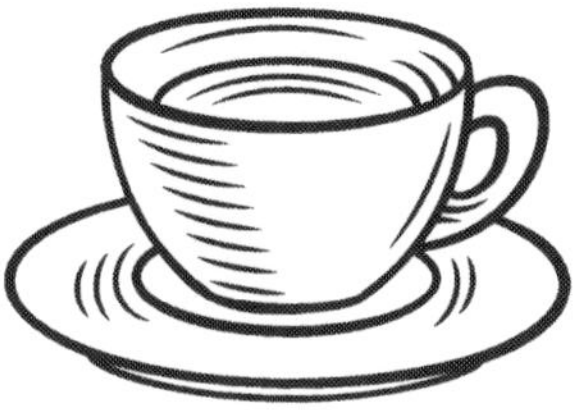

MY STRENGTH IS ... ______________________________

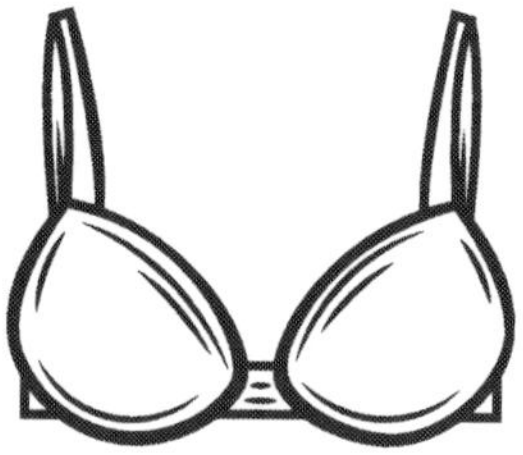

STRENGTH IS ...

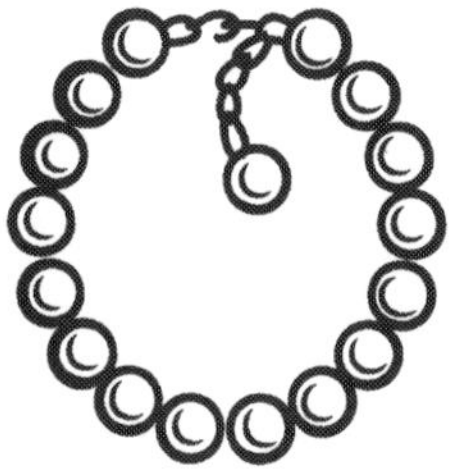

MY STRENGTH IS ... ____________________

MY STRENGTH IS ...

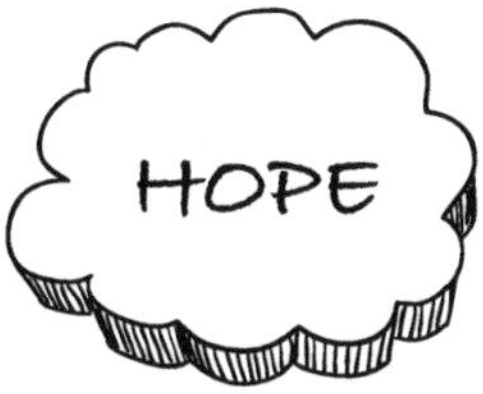
HOPE

MY STRENGTH IS ...

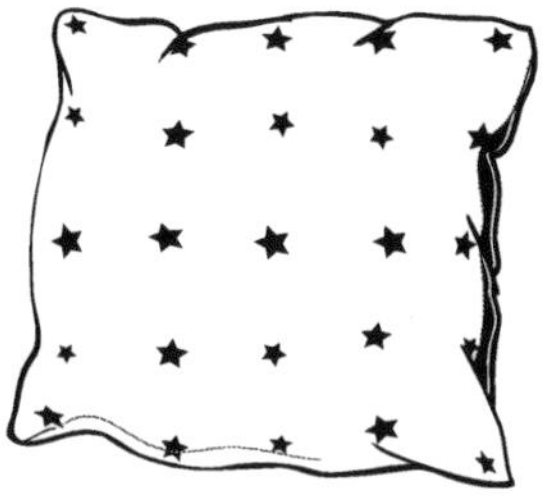

Made in the USA
Monee, IL
26 September 2021

78235714R00059